The 5:2 Fast Diet

Lose Weight Fast Using Our Easy Guide to Intermittent Fasting

by FlatBelly Queens

Published in Great Britain by:

FlatBelly Queens
345 Old Street
London
EC1V 9LE

© Copyright 2016 – Flatbelly Queens

ISBN-13: {978-1533319487}
ISBN-10: {1533319480}

ALL RIGHTS RESERVED. No part of this publication may be reproduced or transmitted in any form whatsoever, electronic, or mechanical, including photocopying, recording, or by any informational storage or retrieval system without express written, dated and signed permission from the author.

Table of Contents

INTRODUCTION:	4
Chapter 1: What is the 5:2 Diet?	8
Chapter 2: Why Do I Want to Follow the 5:2 Diet?	12
Chapter 3: Everything You Need to Know About the 5:2 Diet	21
Chapter 4: How to Handle the Fasting Days	36
Chapter 5: 5:2 Diet Recipes	48
Breakfast	49
Lunch	61
Dinner	76
Chapter 6: What Foods Should I Keep in the House?	90
Conclusion:	98

Introduction:

Losing weight and getting healthy has never been an easy proposition. First, there is so much different advice out there, from calorie restriction to avoiding the foods you love, and none of them sound appealing to you, that you may feel lost and confused. They recommend you cut calories out of your diet, deny yourself, and the result of this is that you often feel hungry, deprived, and irritable. And yet, unless you follow the diet perfectly, every single meal, every single day, you don't manage to lose any weight. Plus, you are probably miserable! Your will power may wane after a few days, and you find yourself falling off the wagon because the diet is almost impossible to stick to. When you are constantly depriving yourself, feeling hungry, and having to exercise will power every second of the day, you feel worn down and irritable. This makes it hard to stick to a plan long enough to make it work. And this is why diets are so hard to follow: constant misery is not the way to live!

But thankfully, there is a solution! And that solution is the 5:2 Diet, which is also known as the intermittent fasting diet. The idea behind the 5:2 diet is that five days a week you are able to eat what you normally would if you are not dieting. For those five days, you do not have to count calories or restrict any foods that you eat. You can still have what you like. You will not feel deprived or feel that you have to cut out foods that you love and enjoy. Then, for two days (which may or may not be consecutive, which is your choice), you fast. But it is not a complete deprivation of food. Instead, on the fasting days, you will eat twenty-five percent of the total calories that you normally eat. For most people, this is 500 calories a day on the fasting days, based on a 2000 calorie diet, which is typical of most people. And you only have to restrict your calories two days per week, not every single day. Because you are not dieting or restricting calories for the majority of your days, it doesn't feel like work and you don't feel like you are depriving yourself, which makes it a much easier diet to stick to. And once you get used to the fasting days, they will come easily to you. Many people report that they have found ways to not feel hungry, even on their fasting days. So, as you see the weight just melt off, you will understand the joys of this diet.

This book will give you all that you need to know to start on the 5:2 Diet plan. The first chapter will describe the 5:2 diet in detail, giving you the basics to get started. Chapter 2 will give you the reasons to follow the 5:2 diet, including some success stories from people who have been where you are now and have had a great deal of success following this diet plan. Seeing that the diet works for normal people will help improve your motivation for the diet and help keep you on track. Chapter 3 will answer all the questions you have about the 5:2 diet, alleviating any questions, confusions, or worries that you have about the 5:2 diet. Chapter 4 will give you a great many suggestions for how to deal with the fast days. After all, this is where you may find yourself struggling, especially at first before you are used to it. This chapter will help teach you to plan for the fasting days, which makes them much easier to stick to. In chapter 5, we will give you some great recipe ideas for you to utilize while following the 5:2 diet plan. Seven breakfast, seven lunch, and seven dinner recipes are included to get you started on making delicious meals, even on your fasting day. Some of them can even be made beforehand, so that you will be prepared when the fasting days come. Then, chapter 6 will give you a good idea of the foods you should keep in your fridge during the 5:2 diet. This is especially helpful on fast days when your caloric intake will be limited. There are even suggestions for snacks under 50 calories. By knowing what foods will help you get through the fasting days, you will have a much easier time sticking to the diet.

Once you are done with this book, you will have all the tools that you need to do the 5:2 diet and start losing weight. You will feel healthier, happier, and thinner as you take control of your weight, your health, and your life! Good luck on your journey, and let's get started!

Chapter 1: What is the 5:2 Diet?

You may have heard the term intermittent fasting. Intermittent fasting means adding in a fast day occasionally to lose weight. The 5:2 diet is considered a diet of intermittent fasting. In the 5:2 diet, you eat normally for five days out of the week and then fast for the other two. But fasting doesn't mean that you eat nothing. Instead, it means a drastic cut in the calories you take in and the kinds of foods you eat.

On the fasting days, you are expected to eat 25 percent of your typical daily caloric intake, or about 500 calories based on the diet of 2000 calories. Some people, including seriously overweight people and men, can go up to 600 calories on these days.

The five non-fasting days are easy: you keep eating what you typically eat. You don't have to cut out foods, count calories, or worry that you are doing something wrong. Those five days you should eat normally. Because of this, there is no need to feel deprived during these days. You can eat what you want and what you like without worry.

It is the other two days, the fasting days, that require a little more planning. Because you will only be eating 500 calories on these days, you need to play out exactly what you are going to eat. If you plan your food well, you will not feel hungry at all. But without planning, you may find yourself going through your calories long before the day is over. Chapter 4 will talk more about how to plan for your fasting days and your eating schedule.

In theory, on the fast days, you can also eat any foods you want, as long as you do not go over your specific calorie limit. However, if you choose to eat all your calories in one meal, the rest of the day will be very difficult.

Because of this, the 5:2 diet has some food recommendations that will allow you to feel full longer and still stay within the limits imposed upon you. This book will give you a good idea of the foods to keep on hand so that you will be able to eat well on the fasting days without feeling hungry. Plus, if you eat high calorie foods, you will waste all your calories very quickly. Although in theory you can eat what you want, you will have more success on your fast days of you stick to lower calorie foods that help fill you up. These include foods that are high in fiber and protein that will help keep you full longer so that you don't struggle on the fast days. Chapter 5 have several recipes that you can use for fast days. Chapter 6 will have a lot of suggestions for foods to eat on fast days to keep you satisfied and to drive away the hunger pangs.

It is that simple. Following the 5:2 intermittent fasting diet will cut your calories by about 3500 calories a week, or a pound per week. You won't feel hungry and you won't feel that you have to constantly deprive of the things that you love. That is the beauty of the diet. You don't have to exercise willpower every second of every day. Five days a week, you will eat normally. It is only the other two days per week that you change up your typical eating habits. The next chapter will discuss the reasons for following the 5:2 diet, including the many health benefits that have been found in people who have followed this diet. It will also answer any questions you have about what you can and cannot do while following this diet. You will find that it is much less restrictive than most diets you could be following today.

Chapter 2: Why Do I Want to Follow the 5:2 Diet?

There are a variety of reasons that you should want to follow the 5:2 diet plan. The obvious one is that you want to lose weight, and this diet has proven to be very successful for people who want to lose weight. It is a diet that has proven to be successful, not only one that can be used for weight loss, butone that people have comfortably made into a lifestyle change that they can stick to. Plus, most of the weight loss was actually fat. Most people who followed intermittent diets did not lose muscle mass when losing weight on them. This is as compared to other diets, where much of the weight lost was muscle mass. If you are not losing fat, but are losing muscle, you are actually doing damage to your body and lowering your metabolism, which makes it more difficult to keep the weight off long term. So, the 5:2 diet has proven to be more effective for weight loss than typical calorie restricted diets and people are able to keep the weight that they lose off.

Besides weight loss, studies on diets that are considered intermittent fasting have shown that there are numerous health benefits to this type of dieting. Although very few studies have been done on the 5:2 diet specifically, diets in this category have been studied extensively, and there are so many benefits for your physical and mental well-being!

First and foremost, when compared to other types of diets, people have been able to maintain their weight loss and their ability to stick to the diet when engaging in intermittent fasting, as compared to calorie-restricted diets. As we have talked about previously, because you are not completely restricting the foods you eat and how often you have to restrict your calories, most people find it easier to stick to. Also, weight loss has either been comparable, or in some cases, even higher, than more traditional diets. Plus, much of the weight lost is found to occur in the belly area. People have lost from 4 to 7 percent of their belly circumference when following these diets. And belly fat is one of the most dangerous types of fat that our body can carry, as it has an effect on the functioning of our vital organs and is said to be a contributing factor to things such as diabetes, heart disease, sleep apnea, colon cancer, high blood pressure, and even premature death. The less belly fat you have, the healthier you will be. So, losing belly fat is one of the best things you can do for overall heath.

Second, many studies on intermittent fasting diets have discovered that it helps improve the problem of insulin resistance. When someone's body is insulin resistant, their body does not respond to the insulin that is supposed to be transporting sugars from the bloodstream and taking it to the rest of the body to fuel the muscles. When the body becomes insulin resistant, diabetes and obesity can be the result. So the fact that intermittent fasting diets help to reduce this problem is a great benefit.

Other health improvements when studies investigated intermittent fasting diets included helping improve the symptoms of seasonal allergies, asthma, hearth arrhythmias, and even menopausal hot flashes! In term of cholesterol, people following an intermittent fasting diet also had a decrease in the triglyceride levels by up to 20 percent! LDL particle size was also increased, which is good. It has been shown that heart disease is more of a problem with people with small LDL particles, and much less of an issue when LDL particle size is higher, so this is definitely something you want to see. Also, the level of leptin in the body was decreased by 40 percent in people following these intermittent fasting diets. Leptin is a protein that helps to regulate fat storage in the body, so with fewer leptin particles, it us harder for the body to store fat. This leads to less weight gain. It will be easier to keep the weight off once you lose it!

Next, following an intermittent fasting diet also decreases the level of C-reactive protein (CRP) in the body. Higher levels of CRP increase inflammation in the body. Chronic inflammation has been shown to be a precursor to many different diseases, including heart disease, some forms of cancer, and even neurodegenerative diseases, such as Alzheimer's and Parkinson's disease. Lowering inflammation in the body has a hugely positive effect on your overall health. Some people have reported that their blood pressure has also been lowed while eating on the 5:2 diet.

And the beautiful thing is that this is a diet that you can adopt for life. Even after you lose the weight that you want, you can modify the diet to maintain your weight loss. When people attain their goal weight, they often choose to switch to a 6:1 diet, meaning that they will fast only one day per week instead of two. In this way, they are able to maintain their weight loss without having to give up anything.

Many people have also reported that following an intermittent fasting plan has helped their mood. They sleep better, have greater stores of energy, can concentrate better, and have an overall sense of well-being. Many have reported less depression and stress in their lives.

Lastly, following an intermittent 5:2 diet plan may even help your body age better. In your body, there are cells that are called free radicals, which have a detrimental effect on your body, causing many of the symptoms that we associate with aging. When the body engages in a fasting cycle, the body is forced to utilize its stores to create energy. When the body burns its own stores for fuel (weight loss), the body will often attack these free radical cells to use as fuel for the body, instead of the typical energy source, the food we eat. When these free radicals are destroyed, our bodies function better and age more gracefully. It also helps for our bodies to handle times of stress more smoothly and easily. Plus, the body will increase their levels of antioxidants calls in the body, which help it to fight against free radicals being formed in the future.

Another way the body is defended against aging is that fasting can inhibit the production of the IGF-1 hormone. Although this hormone may be useful in keeping the body moving, it can also speed up the aging process. When the production of this hormone is slowed down, it enables the body to go into repair mode, so cells are repaired instead of being damaged. This also helps slow down the aging process.

As you can see, there are a great many benefits to using the 5:2 intermittent fasting diet to lose weight. Not only will you lose weight faster (and fat, not muscle), but you will also have a great many health benefits, including decreased risk for diabetes, obesity, heart disease, and even Alzheimer's and Parkinson's! Plus, you won't feel hungry and most people find this diet is a very easy one to follow because you will not feel deprived. You do not have to give up on the foods you love and you don't have to count calories every single day! With all these advantages, is there any doubt about the fact that you want to follow this diet?

Many people have reported feeling better, losing weight, gaining energy, and taking control of their life through the use of the 5:2 intermittent fasting diet plan. Average weight loss has been shown to be anywhere from a few pounds to up to 84 pounds, gaining more lean muscle mass while losing mostly fat, and their energy has increased. Many people also report that they have developed a better relationship with food. By learning to be mindful of what they choose to eat, both on fasting days and non-fasting days, they have paid more attention to what they choose to eat. And though they did not give up the foods that they loved, they were better able to cut down on unconscious eating, which does nothing to help lose weight and is often the biggest reason people gain weight or cannot lose weight. And with the increased energy that they experience with this plan, they are better able to enjoy life more. They have the energy to do the things they have always wanted, but they were not able to do because the weight prevented them from living the life they want. It is amazing the transformation that people following the 5:2 diet plan have experienced. So, why not give it a try for yourself?

One woman lost 31 pounds and was able to stop the yo-yo dieting. She found comfort in the simplicity of the 5:2 diet plan and was able to stick to it, rather than falling off the wagon, gaining the weight back, and trying to diet again. With a plan that she could stick to for life, she found relief from this cycle.

Another woman lost over 20 pounds and found the perfect way to deal with her fasting days by eating lunch and dinner only, as she did not feel hungry in the morning. She was able to manage her fasting days in a way that worked for her without compromising her efforts. And, she is thrilled that she can still eat out at least once a week and still lose weight.

A third person lost 42 pounds and rarely felt hungry on her fast days, even though she ate all her food during one meal at dinner time. If she felt hungry earlier, she would have a very small meal or drink a lot more. She found the perfect way for her to manage her fast days without having to give up anything she really wanted on the other days.

Once people have achieved their weight loss goals, they often will choose to stay on an intermittent diet plan, with a little bit of an adjustment. Instead of doing five days of eating and two days of fasting, which enabled them to lose weight, they change the ratio to six days of eating and one day of fasting (a 6:1 plan). This will help you maintain your weight loss while still receiving the health benefits from intermittent fasting. Plus, you will more easily be able to maintain your new weight because the fasting one day per week will restrict your calories enough that you won't gain back the weight you lose but you won't lose any more. Most people who engage in the 5:2 diet plan see it as something to do for the rest of their lives. It becomes a lifestyle, not just a short-term diet plan.

If you have any questions, the next chapter will answer anything else you may be wondering about the 5:2 diet. After that chapter, you should have all your major questions about the 5:2 diet answered and be ready to dive right in and start a path to better health!

Chapter 3: Everything You Need to Know About the 5:2 Diet

The 5:2 diet seems rather simple, but you may find that you have a lot of questions about what you can and cannot do on the 5:2 diet. This chapter will take the top questions and answer them for you. After you read this, you should feel confident about starting on the 5:2 diet plan. And once you get started, you will realize just how easy and effective this diet really is!

What should I eat on the non-fasting days?

The beauty of the 5:2 diet is that, on non-fasting days, you can eat anything that you want. Out of the seven days of the week, you get to eat your normal foods for five days. You do not have to cut out any specific food or feel restricted by having to count calories. There are no foods that are off-limits, as in some other diet plans. This is what people love about this diet: they do not feel deprived because they have to give up their favorite foods. You can eat anything you like on the days that you are not fasting.

Do I have to count calories on my non-fasting days?

The simple answer is no, you do not have to count calories on the non-fasting days. However, the full answer is that it is a little more complicated than that.

Because the 5:2 diet is based on the idea that you are cutting about 3000-3500 calories per week on the fasting days, which is equivalent to one pound of weight loss, you need to make sure that you are not going overboard on your eating during the non-fasting days.

This means that you don't necessarily need to count calories, but you should try and stay mindful about how much you eat. Large portion sizes, a lot of snacking, or not paying attention to what you eat are all ways that you can sabotage this diet. So, while counting calories is not something that you have to do, it will do better for you to at least pay attention to how much you eat and how often you eat. One reason people tend to gain weight is that they unconscious eat. It is easy to eat too much while vegging out in front of the TV or grabbing a snack every time you get the slightest tummy rumble. By staying mindful of what you are putting in your mouth, even on non-fasting days, you will improve your relationship with food. The typical 2,000 calorie diet at is recommended for most people is the area that you should be shooting for. Some people do choose to count on non-fasting days for greater results, but it is not necessary for most people.

Do my fasting days have to be consecutive, or can I split them up during the week?

You can do either one. Some people find that fasting for two consecutive days (for no longer than 48 hours at a time) is easier for them to maintain. Other people like to split up their fasting days. Do what is easier for you. After all, you need to pick a plan that you will stick to, so whatever you feel is easier for you to do is the way to go.

The nice thing is that you don't have to do the same thing from week to week. The plan requires two fasting days, but you can pick those days that best meet your schedule for that week. Don't be afraid to change the fasting days to make it easier for you to stick to the plan. You can change the fasting days based on your schedule for the week, so you won't have to fast on a day that you have a big social event! The days do not need to be the same from week to week, as long as you get two fasting days in each week.

Typically, a fast goes from dinner one night to breakfast two days hence. So, if your fasting day is Monday, you will fast from after dinner Sunday night until breakfast on Tuesday. If you do your fasting days consecutively, you will go from dinner Sunday night until breakfast Wednesday.

How often should I eat on fasting days?

Most people choose to eat up to three meals on fasting days, but no snacking. However, some of the health benefits are shown to be better if you only eat once or twice a day. The key is to stay under the 500 calorie limit. This is why planning your food intake on fasting days is important: healthy foods go a lot further on the fasting days than non-healthy foods do. We will discuss the different meal plan options in more detail in the chapter on how to handle the fasting days, which is coming up next. You can then choose which meal plan will work best for you.

Is this diet safe for everyone?

Although most people will have good results on the 5:2 intermittent fasting plan and have no problems with following this diet plan, there are some people who should not engage in a fasting plan.

People who should not fast include pregnant women, women who are nursing children, children and teenagers, and anyone with a history of eating disorders. To fast if you fit into one of these categories could be very dangerous for you. Do not attempt this diet if you fall into one of these categories.

As a side note, it is important to check with your doctor before engaging on this diet if you suffer from either Type 1 or Type 2 Diabetes or any chronic medical conditions for which you are being treated. It is possible that fasting will not be healthy for you if you have other major medical issues. If you have any questions, a talk with your doctor should be in order.

For everyone else, cutting calories in such a way is not dangerous and you should have no issues with it. In fact, our ancestors lived on this feasting and fasting approach. When food was available, they ate a lot so that they could get through days when they had to fast because they did not have food available to them. Our bodies evolved to work in this way. This feast and famine cycle was normal for our ancestors, so there is no danger in it. Unless you have a medical condition, there should be no adverse effects for you on the 5:2 diet.

Will my body go into "starvation mode" while on this diet?

When your body goes into starvation mode, your body thinks that food will not be forthcoming for a while, so it tries to conserve energy for future needs so that you do not die. Many people are under the false assumption that depriving yourself of food for one or two days, that will force your body into starvation mode. This means that it will not want to burn the stored fats on your body and will store as much as it can for the future. This is a fallacy, however. It takes several weeks of depriving yourself of calories to get into starvation mode. This is where the 5:2 diet plan has it over other restrictive calorie plans. Because you are only restricting calories for two days per week, your body will not go into starvation mode. On other restrictive plans, on the other hand, where you do restrict calories on a regular basis, there is much more of a chance of this happening. It is not an issue on the 5:2 diet plan.

What is the effect of exercising on the 5:2 diet?

Most people can exercise regularly on the 5:2 diet plan without any adverse effects. In fact, most people can even exercise on fast days without any problems. However, some people choose to save the vigorous workouts for their non-fasting days when they may have more energy. You may need to experiment a little bit to figure out exactly what will work best for you. Just keep in mind that exercising on fast days may be good for you, as long as you don't go at it too hard. Studies have shown that people who exercise while fasting burn more fat than exercising on a non-fasting day.

However, unlike other diets, you do not get to "bank" calories burned from exercise to eat more on the fast days. You still need to stick to your 500 calorie limit, even if you engage in exercise on these days. This way, you will lose more weight and still gain the effects of the intermittent fasting does for your body. After all, your body will utilize its stores to fuel your exercise regimen on fasting days, meaning it will burn more calories per day than if you do not exercise.

On your non-fasting days, it will be helpful to your weight loss efforts to engage in some kind of exercise, especially vigorous exercise if you can. Doing dedicated exercise or just making sure that you stay active on a daily basis will be a great help on your weight loss efforts. Besides exercise, make sure to stay moving. Many fitness devices are on the market now, and you can get one to help you count your steps and activity level throughout the day. Most experts recommend getting in 10,000 steps per day to stay healthy.

No matter what you do, any type of regular exercise will help in your weight loss efforts. As with any diet, staying active will help you achieve your goals faster than sitting down all day. Finding activities that you like to do and find enjoyable will make this easier.

What if I don't feel well?

If you are sick, it is probably best not to fast. Fasting puts some stress on your system, and if you are not feeling well, you may have a more difficult time getting better. So, if you feel symptoms of an illness coming on, move your fasting day until you feel better.

That being said, the first few times you fast, you may have some difficulty adjusting to it. You may feel tired or hungry or your energy levels may wane. This is to be expected. It may be worthwhile to keep a small snack with you if you don't feel well while fasting. After a couple fasting days, however, your body should acclimate to it and you shouldn't have any other issues. Chapter 6 has several snack ideas for when your fasting becomes difficult, including their calorie counts.

Does it have to be five days off and two days on?

No. Some people do change the number of fast days compared to the number of non-fasting days. The most common change is that people will change it to a 4:3 plan, meaning that they fast for three days and eat normally for four. It will speed up your weight loss while still being able to eat the foods you love on non-fasting days. Some people have even changed to an every other day fast, meaning that they fast one day, eat regularly the next, and repeat the cycle. This is a good option if your weight loss stalls or if you want to lose weight faster. Studies have shown that it is not a problem to fast every other day for short periods of time. Also, once you have reached your weight loss goals, many people find that switching to a 6:1 plan helps them maintain the benefits of weight loss and the diet without gaining anything back.

Can I drink alcohol on the 5:2 diet?

On your normal eating days, drinking alcohol is not a problem. Just make sure not to drink to excess, since alcohol contains a lot of calories and may counteract the effects of the fasting days. Remember, moderation is the key here.

As for drinking on fasting days, it is not recommended for two reasons. As already mentioned, alcohol is high in calories, which means that it will consume many of the calories that you are allowed on the fasting days. Second, alcohol is known to produce a spike in the insulin levels, making it harder to manage your blood sugar. This could be especially problematic if you have diabetes and are following this diet. Plus, drinking may cause you to get a little munchy (at least it does for many people), making it difficult to stay under your 500 calorie limit. Drinking alcohol on fasting days will be discussed in more depth in the chapter on how to handle the fasting days.

How much weight can I lose on the 5:2 diet?

How much weight you will lose on this diet can vary greatly. First, it depends on how much you have to go to reach your goal weight. Also, the amount of weight you lose can be dependent on your age, your level of activity, and even what you choose to eat on your non-fasting days. Although this diet does not require you to count calories on the five days that you do not fast, by making sure not to overeat or going crazy on these days, you will lose more weight. Plus, if you exercise regularly, you will lose weight faster than if you do not, as you will be burning more calories than if you lead a sedentary lifestyle.

These facts are true for any weight loss program. Plus, you will probably drop some weight very quickly at the beginning of the diet, but your weight loss may slow down as your body becomes more acclimated to the 5:2 plan. As for total weight loss, people have reported losing a few pounds to up to about 85 pounds! It all depends on where you are on your weight loss journey.

We recommend that, besides keeping track of the weight you lose, it is also advisable to do regular body measurements so that you can see your actual progress. Taking measurements of your chest, waist, and hips will help you get a better, clearer account of how your body is changing, rather than just relying on weight as your only milestone. Sometimes weight loss isn't just seen on the scale, but is also seen in the body measurements.

What if I stop losing weight?

Keep in mind that how much weight you lose may change from week to week as your body acclimates to this diet. You may lose more one week than the next. Also, there is some natural fluctuation in weight from day to day.

However, if you go more than three weeks without any weight loss, there could be a few things that may be happening:

> First, your body may be re-proportioning itself. Muscle is denser than fat, meaning that, if you are developing more muscle, you could be getting thinner without seeing any change on the scale. This is why it is useful to take body measurements. If you haven't lost any weight, re-measure your chest, waist, and hips to see if you are getting skinnier. Or, you can try on a pair of pants. If they are looser, your body is going through some changes that aren't showing on the scale yet. Stick to the plan and you will start to see changes in your weight soon.
> Second, you may be eating too much on your non-fasting days. Cut back just a little bit. Reducing potion sizes is usually the best way to accomplish this. Some people choose to count calories if they see the scale stuck. You may be surprised to find out how much you do eat on a non-fasting day. Remember, for most adults, a 2,000 calorie diet is what is recommended. It doesn't mean that you have to restrict what foods you

like, it just means that you should eat a little less of them. After all, moderation is healthy.

On the other end of the spectrum, you could be under-eating on your non-fasting days and your body is feeling starved. If this is happening, your body will enter starvation mode where it will horde all the calories it can and you will not gain weight. Make sure you are eating enough on your normal days. Although this is less likely, it can still be a problem. Try tracking your non-fast day foods for a few days to see if you are eating too little. Remember, 2000 calories is the goal for most people. IF you have been too restrictive of food on your non-fasting days for a few weeks, this could be an issue. Up your calorie intake a little bit on non-fasting days.

Look at specific calories you are taking in on your non-fasting days, specifically what you are drinking. Things such as juices, lattes, smoothies, and alcohol can contain a lot more calories than you think, and it may be beneficial to reduce or cut them from your diet. A lot of drinks are very high in calories, which many people don't know. A small latte can contain 200 calories! By being aware of this fact, you can make the conscious choice about how many calories you drink. Keep in mind that drinking your calories does not make you feel full, whereas eating the same amount will. This means you may take in many more calories when you drink high calorie things than if you eat them.

Exercise more. As we've already talked about, getting regular exercise will boost your weight loss efforts. Even just getting up and taking a short walk every hour or two will help you lose weight. Staying active will help you burn more calories, which leads to more weight loss.

Your body may need a little bit of a kick start. Try upping your fast days to three days per week. A 4:3 diet cycle for a couple weeks could help restart your ability to lose. Then you can move back to the 5:2 ratio to keep your weight loss going.

Is this just a diet plan, or can I stay on it for a long time?

Many people have made the 5:2 diet a lifestyle change. Once their body is used to eating and fasting, they find that it is easy to stick to and they feel good. Some people, once they have reached their desired weight, will shift to a 6:1 plan, fasting only one day per week, in order to maintain the weight loss without losing anything more. This will help with weight loss maintenance while still gaining and reaping the benefits of fasting, as they have been described. No matter what you choose to do, the 5:2 plan can be a weight loss and lifestyle plan, not just a short-term diet. And because you don't feel deprived, you will be able to stick with it for a lifetime!

Now that you have all your basic questions answered, let's move on to discuss in detail how to deal with your fasting days. These days are the bread and butter of your eating plan and the ones that people new to this diet struggle with. With the information in the next chapter, you will gain a great understanding about how to manage your fasting days successfully without feeling hungry or deprived.

Chapter 4: How to Handle the Fasting Days

Fasting days are the major part of the 5:2 diet. This is where your calorie restriction comes in. Instead of feeling deprived every single day on this diet, you are only required to restrict your calories for two days per week. The other five days, you can eat as you normally would.

On the fasting days, you are to limit your calories to

approximately 500 calories per day. Some people can go as high as 600 calories, but that should be your upper limit. In this book, I regularly refer to the 500 calorie limit as the standard, as this is what most people follow. Some people recommend that women stay at the 500 calorie limit, while men, who tend to burn more calories in a day, can go up to 600. Also, people who weigh more may do better with the 600 calorie limit than with people who are closer to their goal weight.

The key to getting through the fasting days is to plan. If you have a plan for what you are going to eat and when, you will be able to stave off hunger. The key is choosing foods that are low calorie, yet delicious and filling so that you do not feel hungry. The next chapter will give you 21 recipes for you to start your fasting days- seven breakfasts, seven lunch, and seven dinner- so that you will have a place to begin.

Of course, on fasting days, you can eat whatever foods you want. You just don't want to go over the calorie limit. That is why it may be in your best interests to plan your foods beforehand and to avoid high calorie foods. After all, if you have all 500 calories at breakfast, you will be hungry the rest of the day. But, if you may a healthy, filling, low calorie breakfast (approximately 100 calories), then you can still eat well the rest of the day without feeling deprived.

Keep in mind, the first few times you fast, you may find it difficult to stick to the plan. Your body will need to adjust to the restriction in calories. You may find that you feel tired or lethargic. I recommend that people keep a snack on hand if they start to not feel well during the first couple fasts. Once you are used to it, these feelings should go away. In fact, after a few times, you may feel freer on the fast days. After all, food will not be what you are concerning yourself with.

The first thing you need to be aware of is that a fast day is actually 36 hours, not 24. Let's take an example: let's say your fast day is on Monday. On Sunday night, when you finish dinner, say 7:30 PM, you are done eating for that night and the next day, except for your 500 calories. It is counterproductive to sneak in a midnight snack. So, your fast will go from 7:30 PM on Sunday night until breakfast time on Tuesday morning. If you do your two fast days in a row, you would start your fast at 7:30 PM on Sunday and go through breakfast time on Wednesday morning.

The second thing is to choose how you will do your meals. There are several options available to you. Some people choose to have one meal where they eat all of their calorie allotment. Most people, however, have a difficult time with this plan because they feel hungry. If you eat your 500 calories at 8 AM, you will go until 8 AM the next morning without anything to eat. And if you choose to eat your one meal at dinner time, you will have gone 24 hours without eating, which makes the plan more difficult to stick with (although some people have found this option the easiest one). Although some people prefer this, it is not necessarily recommended. It may be easier for you to cheat if you are feeling deprived, so it ends up being counterproductive to the idea of the diet.

The second options, which is what most people do, is to split their calories between two main meals, one in the morning and one in the middle of the afternoon or early evening. The advantage to this is that each meal will be approximately 250-300 calories, giving you more options for what to eat. The biggest disadvantage of this is that you may still suffer some hunger pangs later in the evening or in between your two meals. This could work well, though, if you know when your hungriest times are. For example, I usually find that I feel the hungriest between breakfast and lunch, but have no problem with hunger in the evenings. So, this would be a good option for me. However, if you are a night eater, you may want to change the times that you eat your two meals, such as lunch and dinner time. Many people who often skip breakfast find that this is a better way for them to handle a two meal fast.

The third option is to eat three meals. This gives you the option to split up your calories in many different ways. Most experts recommend keeping breakfast to under 100 calories, then allotting 200-250 calories to each lunch and dinner. This will allow you to keep a regular meal schedule, one that your body is probably most used to, and keep yourself from being hungry throughout the day.

The last option is to have several small meals, say of 100 calories each. Some people like the idea that they can eat more often, which helps keep hunger at bay and helps them deal with the psychological issues that may come up when they approach a fast day. Some people struggle with the concept of having to regulate their meals in such a way, and find that small snacks throughout the day works best for them.

One of the most important keys here is to not snack in between (unless you are choosing to have 5 small meals, for example). Too often we are used to feeling hungry and automatically grabbing a snack before we even realize what we are doing. It requires a little bit of mindfulness to really get through the fasting days because you will need to stop yourself from the subconscious munching that is probably one of the biggest causes of weight gain in our culture.

The key here is to figure out what works best for you so that fast days aren't seen as difficult or as a chore. Once you have gotten used to fasting, you will find out what works best for you and work out a specific plan that you can stick to. Most people find that, once they have found the plan they like, they don't feel hungry on their fast days.

One thing to keep in mind is that, oftentimes, people eat because they think they are hungry, but, in reality, they are actually thirsty. Study after study have shown that most of our culture is dehydrated, but they cannot distinguish between the need for food and the need for drink. That is why I recommend that, when you feel hungry on the fast days (and on non-fast days too, if you are trying to be mindful about your food), you drink. But what you choose to drink is something to be careful of here. There are plenty of things that we drink that are chock full of calories that you may not even realize. Let's first talk about some drinks that you should avoid on fast days, then we will talk about things that are good to drink when that hunger urge hits you.

Fruit juices, soda, lattes, and flavored drinks are often chock full of calories and sugar. Many dieters are amazed that, when they look up their favorite drink from their coffee shop of choice, they contain hundreds of calories!

They had no idea how much damage that morning frap or latte was costing them and contributing to their weight gain! Even regular coffee, if you add sugar and creamer, can have a lot of calories that you may not even think about. So, if you are drinking coffee, it is best to go with straight black, as this has no calories to speak of. If you have to have something in your coffee, a little splash of milk will add a negligible amount of calories, but far less than cream and sugar. Before choosing a drink, make sure that you aren't adding any calories that you don't know are there.

The other thing that you probably want to avoid on fasting days is alcohol, although this isn't an absolute. Some people can drink a little alcohol on fast days and have no issues. However, it is important to keep in mind that alcohol can be very high in calories (cutting into how much you can eat because, yes, these calories count!), and that alcohol can spike your insulin levels, giving you a sugar high and crash that could make dealing with fast days even more difficult for you. When you spike your insulin levels, you will have a great deal of energy for a short period of time, but the crash after can be very difficult to deal with, making you crave food more than usual to get it back up. This leads to a cycle that can sabotage your diet efforts. It is something that is best avoided on fast days.

Now that you have examined whether your go-to drink is full of calories (and maybe had to get rid of it on fast days), let's look at some things that are good for you to drink. These can be your go-to drinks when you feel a little bit of hunger. Chances are you are probably more thirsty than hungry anyway.

First, you should make sure to drink plenty of water. Many dieticians recommend drinking a glass of water before every meal, and this may be especially helpful on fasting days, although it is good advice for every day. Your stomach will be a little more full before you start eating, making you want to eat less and helping you to feel full faster. Plus, you can keep a bottle of water with you at all times to sip on. Conventional wisdom says that you should drink about 64 ounces of water a day, but your personal needs may be a little more or a little less.

Other good beverages that are good to have on fast days include black coffee (and we have already discussed why it needs to be black), any kind of teas, flavored water (as long as it is calorie free), and seltzer. Basically, anything no calorie or low calorie is good to have.

Let me add one thing here. Many people give up sugary sodas and go to diet sodas as a substitute. Since they are all no calorie or almost no calorie, this can be a good switch for you. However, studies have shown that drinking diet sodas can make you crave more sugary and fatty foods. This is because artificial sweeteners may still cause the spike in blood sugar that is often seen with sugary drinks. This makes you crave more food as your blood sugar quickly drops and your energy level wanes. You may want to examine whether this is the case for you, and if it is, if it is something that you can deal with. Diet sodas aren't off limits on fast days, but see if you can get a handle for how they affect your body. You may be surprised by the results.

Now that you know when you should eat and what you should eat, let's talk a little bit about the foods that are good to have on fast days. After all, planning for your fasting days are the best way to succeed. If you have made plans to alleviate hunger, you will be less likely to cheat. And once you start to see results, you will swear by these days. But they can be intimidating at first to get used to, so let's talk a little bit about a plan.

It will be easier to tackle fast days if you have a plan for what you will eat. So, let's take an example so you can see how to do it. We will choose a three meal option.

Sit down the day before your fast and make sure that you have all the ingredients that you need to prepare the foods that you will eat. That way, you won't have to go to the store at the last minute. The final chapter in this book will give you a hint of things to keep in the pantry for fast days (and that may be helpful for non-fast days too), so you will not be caught off guard. Some people even choose to make some of the recipes beforehand so that, on fast days, their food will already be prepared, making it easier to stick to.

Make a meal plan:

For breakfast, scrambled eggs and mushrooms (see recipes) sound good, and at 78 calories, it is the perfect start. It's well under 100 calorie limit, and the protein in the eggs will be filling. You can even add a cup of spinach to the eggs and mushrooms for just an additional 7 calories! So, we start the day with 86 calories.

For lunch, you have made some Alkalizing green soup ahead of time, for 182 calories. You add a piece of low-calorie wheat bread for 40 calories, bringing your lunch total to 222 calories. Total for the day, 308 calories.

For dinner, you make some Cacciatore chicken, for a total of 171 calories. For the day, you have eaten 479 calories. During the day, you have had plenty of water, a cup of coffee with a little milk, and a cup of tea in the evening. You don't feel the need to snack, and you don't feel too hungry, even though you have only had approximately 500 calories (with the milk in your coffee). Now, you are done eating until breakfast the next morning.

By making this plan, there is no question about how much you are eating and when you should be eating. You know that you have everything you need to cook in the house, and you even prepared the soup the weekend before when you had more time to cook. This way, you felt prepared to handle your fast day effectively! This is the best way to handle it.

In general, the foods that are best for fast days include those that are high in protein and fiber, as these will keep you feeling fuller longer. This includes lean meats, fish, and vegetables. Veggies are especially great because they can give you that full feeling with their high fiber content, but they cost very few calories. If you feel the need to snack on a fast day, veggies are a good option because they will not typically take away many of the calories you have allocated to your meals. Other low-calorie snacking options are discussed in Chapter 6.

Many people ask how they can track their calories on fast days (and maybe even non-fasting days). There are plenty of online calorie trackers or apps for your tablet or smart phone that will help you do this quickly and easily. One of the most popular is My Fitness Pal, but there are plenty of options available out there where you can track your calorie count for free, so figure out what works best for you.

As you can see, planning for fast days is the key to success. If it is your fast day and you are unprepared, it will be harder to stick to it. But, if you have made a grocery list, planned out your menu, and made sure that everything you need is already in the house, you will be ready to conquer the day without any issues! And since it is only two days per week, it is not overwhelming to plan, as it may be on some other diets which require a meal plan for every day and every meal. The next chapter contains 21 recipes for you to use on fast days to help keep your calorie count low and still enjoy the day. Of course, once you have tried these, there are plenty of other options available to you on the internet and in many different books, but you can get started here and takes weeks to try them all! The last chapter, then, will describe what you should keep in your kitchen for fast days. By stocking your pantry with healthy foods, you may even find yourself eating them on days that you do not have to fast. If the food is delicious and easy to prepare, you may start eating better all week long!

Chapter 5: 5:2 Diet Recipes

This chapter contains recipes to follow and eat on the fast days. The calorie counts and servings are listed for each recipe so that there will be no guessing when it comes to how much you are eating. Seven breakfast, seven lunch, and seven dinner recipes are included. It is important to note here that many of these recipes are using weight measures to measure food (many in grams). This is to make sure that the foods are made exactly so that the calorie counts are right. After all, a few calories here and a few calories there, and you may be getting way more than you expected to. So, it is worthwhile to invest in a good digital kitchen scale that measures in grams for this diet. This will assure that you have the exact measurements and are not going over your counts.

These recipes are easy to make (many of them you can make beforehand) and are delicious. This is important because, if you are still eating well on fast days, you will be able to stick to it. Give these recipes a try. They will make fast days go much more smoothly.

Breakfast

Banana Oat Muffins

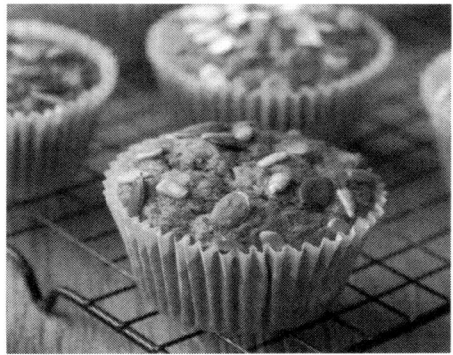

Makes 12

Calories per muffin: 219

Preparation time: 15 minutes

Cooking time: 20–25 minutes

Ingredients
  100g rolled oats

  50g whole wheat flour

  150g plain white flour

  2 tsp baking powder

  1 tsp bicarbonate of soda

  ¼ tsp salt

  75g muscovado sugar

  4 large very ripe bananas, mashed

  1 large egg, beaten

  4 tbsp. light olive oil

  2 tbsp. pumpkin or sunflower seeds or a mix

- Preheat the oven to 180°C/350°F/Gas mark 4. Line a 12-hole muffin tin with paper cases.

- Mix together the oats (keeping a tablespoon aside

for the topping), flours, baking powder, bicarbonate of soda, salt and sugar.

- Mix together the mashed bananas, egg and oil and then pour into the dry oat and flour mix and fold together.

- Spoon into the prepared muffin cases and scatter the top of each muffin with the reserved oats and the seeds. Bake for 20–25 minutes, until brown and slightly springy to touch.

Kiwi, Greek yogurt and blueberries

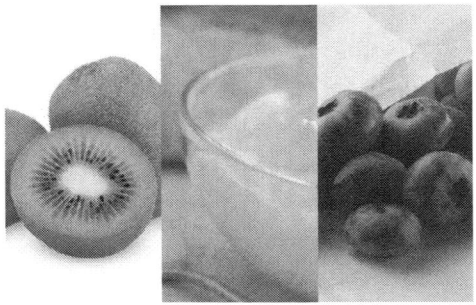

95 Calories per serving

Ingredients

1 chopped kiwi

3 tbsp. fat-free Greek yogurt

50g blueberries

- A few tablespoons of yogurt, a handful of blueberries and some chopped and peeled kiwi can go a long way to make this sweet start to the day which is low in calories but not in flavor! Combine together in a bowl or blitz in a food processor for a quick yogurt smoothie on the move!

Scrambled egg and mushrooms

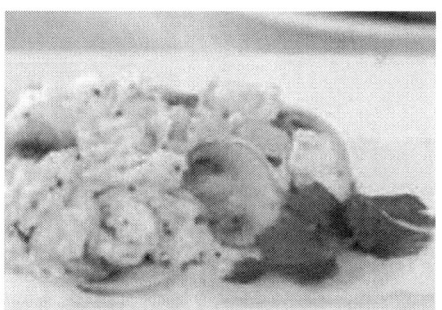

Ingredients

1 medium egg

100g fresh mushrooms chopped

Total calories = 91 for 1 serving

- Scrambled egg is ideal for breakfast as the protein in the egg will keep you full until lunch time - just avoid adding milk and butter and make with only one egg. Mixed with a handful of fresh mushrooms, this combo gives the eggs more texture and flavor and bulks it out a bit. Cook the eggs in a non-stick frying pan without oil. Once the eggs are almost cooked, add the mushrooms (and leafy greens) until the eggs are cooked. You can add some leafy greens such as spinach to increase the fiber in this meal.

Porridge with blueberry compote

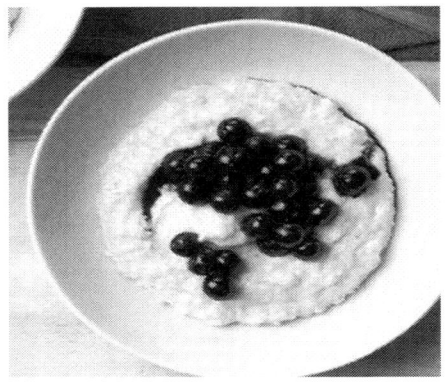

Makes 2 Servings

168 calories per serving

Ingredients

6 tbsp. porridge oats

Just under ½ x 200ml tub 0% fat Greek-style yogurt

½ x 350g pack frozen blueberries

1 tsp honey (optional)

Method

- Put the oats in a non-stick pan with 400ml water and cook over the heat, stirring occasionally for about 2 minutes until thickened. Remove from the heat and add a third of the yogurt.

- Meanwhile, tip the blueberries into a pan with 1 tbsp. water and the honey if using and gently poach until the blueberries have thawed and they are tender, but still holding their shape.
- Spoon the porridge into bowls, top with the remaining yogurt and spoon over the blueberries.

Baked eggs with spinach & tomato

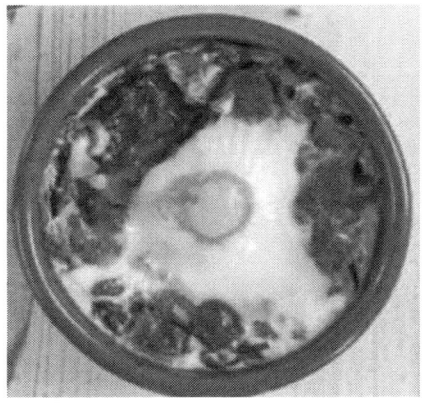

Makes 4 servings

114 calories per serving

Ingredients
- 100g bag spinach
- 400g can chopped tomatoes
- 1 tsp chili flakes
- 4 eggs

Method

- Heat oven to 350 F. Put the spinach into a colander, then pour over a kettle of boiling water to wilt the leaves. Squeeze out excess

water and divide between 4 small ovenproof dishes.
- Mix the tomatoes with the chili flakes and some seasoning, then add to the dishes with the spinach. Make a small well in the center of each and crack in an egg. Bake for 12-15 mins or more depending on how you like your eggs. Serve with crusty bread, if you like. Just make sure to count the calories on the bread!

Banana Berry Smoothie

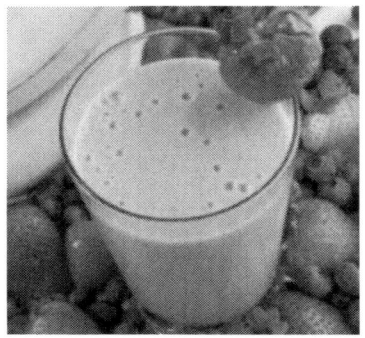

Serves 2

127 Calories each

Ingredients
½ cup blueberries

½ cup raspberries

1 medium sliced banana (ripe)

½ cup apple juice (unsweetened)

1 ½ teaspoons honey

1/8 teaspoon ground cinnamon or cinnamon powder

½ cup ice

Directions

- Simply add the ingredients in a blender and pulse a few times until the fruit is all chopped up. Stir well and then blend the mixture until smooth and drinkable.

Spinach and Egg Whites Omelet

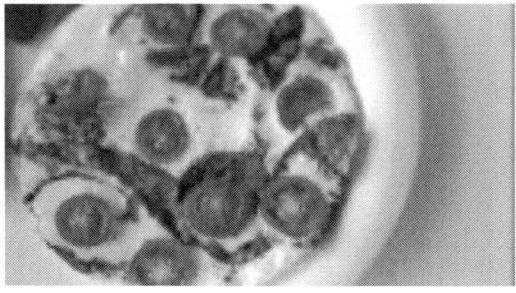

Total Calories: 80 for 1 serving

Ingredients:
- 3 Egg Whites
- 1/2 cups Spinach, finely chopped
- 3 Cherry Tomatoes, thinly sliced
- 1 TSP Grated Parmesan Cheese
- Pinch of Pepper

Directions:

- Whisk together egg whites, then mix in the spinach and tomatoes. Pour into a skillet that is (lightly) sprayed with cooking spray. Add the pepper. Cook to your liking, then sprinkle the Parmesan just before serving.

Lunch

Leak, Potato, and Pea Soup

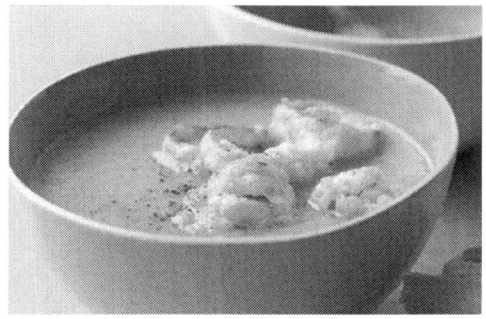

134 calories per serving.

Makes 6 servings

Ingredients

2 large leeks (about 500g), well washed

1 onion, peeled and chopped

30g butter

2 vegetable stock pots or cubes

1 large potato (about 250g) peeled and chopped

100g peas

For the garnish:

1 medium egg white

A pinch of saffron threads

1 level tbsp. plain flour

Oil, for frying

Note: Use a fork to dip the leeks in the batter and a draining spoon to take them out of the hot oil. Add some cream to make it extra special.

Method

- Set aside a 10cm piece of leek for the garnish. Slice the rest of the leek and cook in a large pan with the onion, in the butter, until softened – about 10 minutes. Pour in 1 liter water and add the stock pots/cubes. Bring to the boil, add the potato and simmer for 10 minutes. Add the peas and cook for another 10 minutes.
- Meanwhile, put the egg white in a small bowl, add the saffron strands and leave to infuse. Slice the reserved leek and put the separated rings in cold water. Whisk the egg white, then whisk in the flour and seasoning to make a smooth batter.
- Blend the soup in a food processor until smooth (or keep it lumpy if you prefer). Season and reheat if necessary.
- Heat some oil in a small pan, drain and dry the leek rings, then dip them in batter and fry until golden and crunchy. Drain on kitchen paper.

Pour the soup into bowl, add crispy leek rings and seasoning.

Asian Chicken Salad

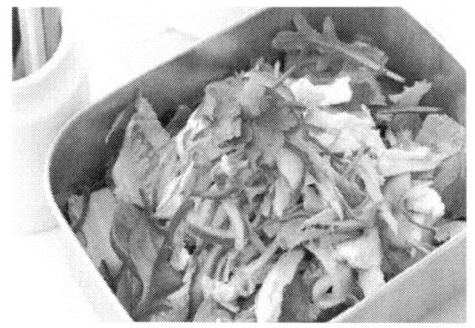

Makes 2 Servings
109 calories each serving

Ingredients
1 boneless, skinless chicken breast
1 tbsp. fish sauce
Zest and juice ½ lime (about 1 tbsp.)
1 tsp caster sugar
100g bag mixed salad leaves
Large handful coriander, roughly chopped
¼ red onion, thinly sliced
½ chili, deseeded and thinly sliced
¼ cucumber, halved lengthways, sliced

Method

- Cover the chicken with cold water, bring to the boil, and then cook for 10 mins. Remove from the pan and tear into shreds. Stir together the fish sauce, lime zest, juice and sugar until sugar dissolves.

- Place the leaves and coriander in a container, then top with the chicken, onion, chili and cucumber. Place the dressing in a separate container and toss through the salad when ready to eat.

Beetroot & squash salad with horseradish cream

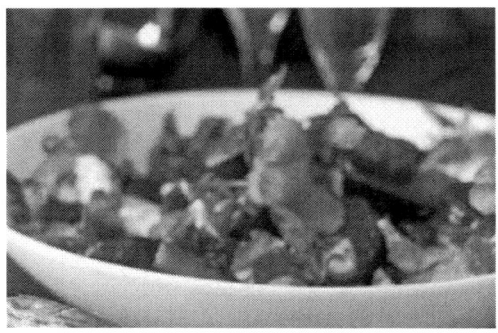

Makes 12 servings
171 calories per serving

Ingredients
1kg raw beetroot
6 red onion
1¼kg large butternut squash, peeled and deseeded
2 tbsp. red wine vinegar
1 tbsp. soft brown sugar
50ml olive oil

For the horseradish cream
175ml soured cream
3 tbsp. creamed horseradish
Juice 1 lemon
85g watercress, large stalks removed

Method

- Heat oven to 350 F. Peel the beetroot and cut each into 8 wedges. Cut the onions and

butternut squash into roughly the same size. Spread out in a large roasting tin. Mix the vinegar and sugar until dissolved, then whisk in the oil. Pour over the vegetables, toss and roast for 40-45 mins until charred and soft, stirring halfway through cooking.
- To make the horseradish cream, mix together the soured cream, horseradish, lemon juice and some seasoning.
- To serve, put the roasted veg in a large bowl or on a platter, followed by the watercress, then drizzle over the horseradish cream. Serve warm or cold.

Alkalizing green soup

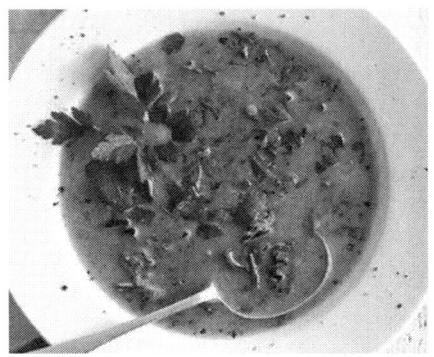

Makes 2 servings
182 calories per serving

Ingredients
500ml stock, made by mixing 1 tbsp. bouillon powder and boiling water in a jug
1 tbsp. sunflower oil
2 garlic cloves, sliced
Thumb-sized piece ginger, sliced
½ tsp ground coriander
3cm/1in piece fresh turmeric root, peeled and grated, or ½ tsp ground turmeric
Pinch of pink Himalayan salt
200g courgettes, roughly sliced
85g broccoli
100g kale, chopped
1 lime, zested and juiced
Small pack parsley, roughly chopped, reserving a few whole leaves to serve

Method

- Put the oil in a deep pan, add the garlic, ginger, coriander, turmeric and salt, fry on a medium heat for 2 mins, and then add 3 tbsp. water to give a bit more moisture to the spices.
- Add the courgettes, making sure you mix well to coat the slices in all the spices, and continue cooking for 3 mins. Add 400ml stock and leave to simmer for 3 mins.
- Add the broccoli, kale and lime juice with the rest of the stock. Leave to cook again for another 3-4 mins until all the vegetables are soft.
- Take off the heat and add the chopped parsley. Pour everything into a blender and blend on high speed until smooth. It will be a beautiful green with bits of dark speckled through (which is the kale). Garnish with lime zest and parsley.

Prawn & pink grapefruit noodle salad

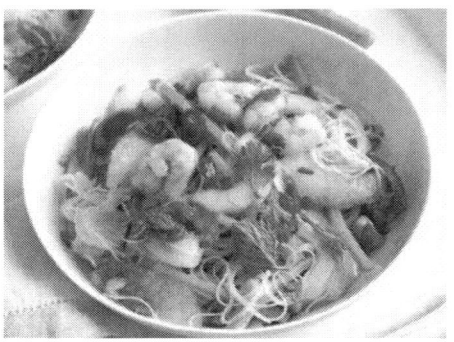

Makes 6 servings
228 calories per serving

Ingredients
200g thin rice noodle (vermicelli)
12 cherry tomato, halved
1 tbsp. fish sauce
Juice 1 lime
2 tsp palm sugar or soft brown sugar
1 large red chili, ½ diced, ½ sliced
2 pink grapefruit, segmented
½ cucumber, peeled, deseeded and thinly sliced
2 carrot, cut into matchsticks
3 spring onion, thinly sliced
400g cooked large prawn
Large handful mint, leaves picked
Large handful coriander, leaves picked

Method

- Put the noodles in a bowl, breaking them up a little, and cover with boiling water from the

kettle. Leave to soak for 10 mins until tender. Drain, rinse under cold running water, and then leave the noodles to drain thoroughly.
- In the same bowl, lightly squash the cherry tomatoes – we used the end of a rolling pin. Stir in the fish sauce, lime juice, sugar and diced chili. Taste for the right balance of sweet, sour and spicy – adjust if necessary.
- Toss through the noodles, then add all the remaining ingredients, except the sliced chili. Season and give everything a good stir, then divide the noodle salad between 6 serving dishes and sprinkle over the chili before serving.

Potato & paprika tortilla

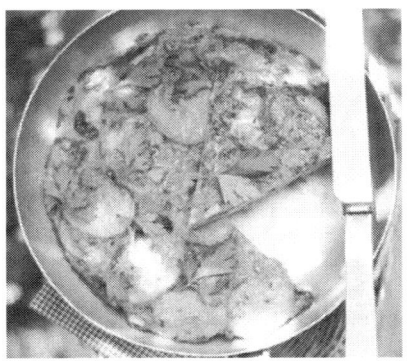

Makes 4 servings
241 calories per serving

Ingredients
3 tbsp. olive oil
250g new potato, ends trimmed, thickly sliced
1 small onion, halved and sliced
2 garlic clove, chopped
½ tsp smoked paprika
½ tsp dried oregano or 3 tbsp. chopped parsley, plus a few extra leaves to garnish (optional)
6 large egg

Method

- Heat the oil in a deep 20cm non-stick frying pan. Fry the potatoes, onion and garlic for 10 mins until tender. Stir in the paprika and fry for 1 min more.
- Beat the dried or fresh herbs into the eggs with seasoning, then pour into the pan. Stir a

couple of times as the egg starts to set on the bottom of the pan, then leave alone to cook slowly over a very low heat for 10 mins until set, except for the very top.
- Carefully slide the tortilla onto a plate. Slide back into the pan, with the uncooked top now on the bottom, and cook for 1-2 mins more. Garnish with parsley, if using, wrap in foil and serve warm or chilled.

Mexican Chicken Soup

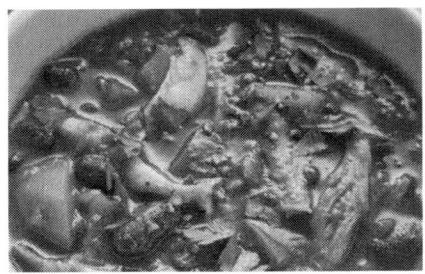

361 calories

SERVES 4 • READY IN 45 MINUTES

Ingredients

4 chicken drumsticks
2 shallots, peeled and roughly chopped
1 carrot, peeled and roughly chopped
1 liter water
1x400g can chopped tomatoes
300ml passata
1 green pepper, deseeded and chopped
1 red chili, deseeded and finely chopped
2 cloves garlic, peeled and crushed
1 tsp dried mixed herbs
1 tsp paprika
1 tsp smoked paprika
½ tsp turmeric
½ tsp ground cumin
1 tsp mild chili powder
1x400g can black beans, drained
1x400g can kidney beans, drained
30g (very large handful) flat leaf parsley, chopped
Salt and freshly ground black pepper

Method

- Place the chicken drumsticks, shallots and carrot in a large saucepan. Pour over the water and bring up to a simmer. Cook for 20 minutes, then remove the chicken drumsticks with a slotted spoon and set aside to cool.
- Add the chopped tomatoes, passata, green pepper, chili and garlic and bring back up to simmering point. Add the dried herbs, paprika, smoked paprika, turmeric, cumin and chili powder, then simmer gently for 30 minutes.
- Remove the skin from the drumsticks and pull as much chicken as possible off the bone. Shred the chicken meat and return it to the pan, along with the black beans and kidney beans for the last 5 minutes of cooking. Remove from the heat and stir in the parsley. Season generously with salt and pepper.

Dinner

Chinese Vegetable Chow Mein

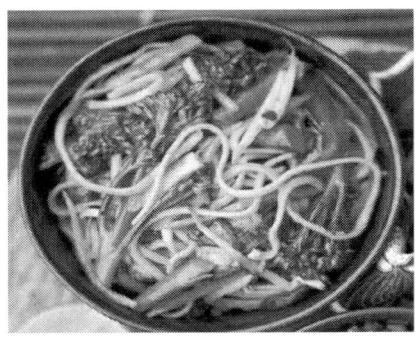

Makes 5 servings

170 Calories per Serving

Ingredients
- 2 tbsp. groundnut or vegetable oil
- 125g packet oyster mushrooms, sliced
- 1 red pepper, deseeded and sliced
- 125g packet tender stem broccoli, cut into pieces
- 1 carrot, peeled and sliced
- 1 tbsp. soy sauce

1 tbsp. rice vinegar

1-2 tbsp. oyster sauce

300g ready-to-use medium egg noodles

1 lime, to serve

Note: If you want to add some meat to this dish, we'd recommend cooked chicken

Method

- Heat the oil in a wok or large frying pan. Add the veg and cook for 2-3 mins. Pour in the soy sauce, vinegar and oyster sauce. Add the noodles to the pan and heat through.
- Serve immediately with some lime squeezed over the top.

Paillard of chicken with lemon & herbs

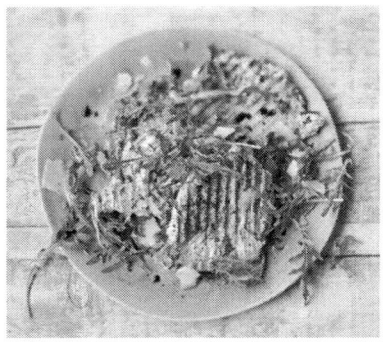

Makes 2 Servings

240 calories per serving

Ingredients
6 skinless chicken breasts

2 tbsp. olive oil

1/2 tbsp. balsamic vinegar

140g bag rocket

25g Parmesan

Lemon wedges

For the marinade
2 garlic cloves

3 rosemary sprigs, leaves finely chopped

6 sage leaves, finely shredded

Zest 1 lemon and juice of ½

3 tbsp. olive oil

Method

- Place each chicken breast between 2 sheets of cling film or baking parchment. Use a meat mallet or rolling pin to bash each piece of chicken – flatten out to an even layer about 0.5cm thick. Transfer to a dish.
- To make the marinade, crush the garlic with a good pinch of salt using a pestle and mortar. Add the rosemary and sage, and give everything a good pounding. Stir through the lemon zest and juice, olive oil and some ground black pepper. Pour the marinade over the chicken, ensuring that it's well coated. Cover and chill for at least 2 hrs.
- Heat the barbecue. Once the flames have died down, spread the coals out to an even layer. Cook the chicken for 1-2 mins each side. Transfer to a board and leave to rest for a few mins.
- Meanwhile, pour the oil and balsamic vinegar into a large bowl. Add the rocket and some seasoning. Toss together, then shave over the Parmesan. Serve the salad with the chicken, with lemon wedges to squeeze over.

Cacciatore chicken

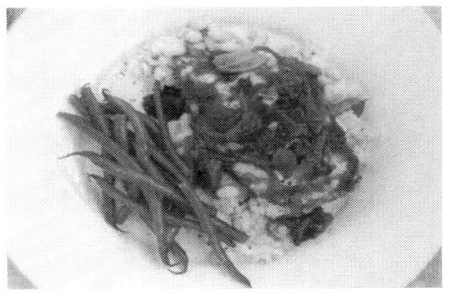

Makes 4 servings

171 calories per serving

Ingredients
1 onion, sliced

2 garlic clove, sliced

1 tsp olive oil

400g can chopped tomato

2 tbsp. chopped rosemary leaves

4 chicken breast

Small handful basil leaves

Favorite seasonal vegetables, to serve (optional)

Method

- Fry the onion and garlic in the oil until softened. Add the tomatoes, rosemary and seasoning, and cook for 10-15 mins until thickened.
- Heat oven to 350 F. Put the chicken on a baking tray, top with the sauce and bake for 15-20 mins until cooked through. Serve scattered with basil, with your favorite veg, if you like.

Spiced pepper pilafs

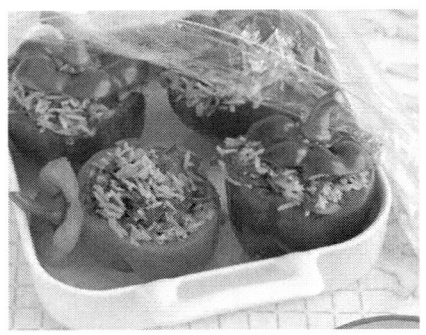

Makes 8 servings

209 calories per serving

Ingredients
1 tbsp. vegetable oil

1 onion, finely chopped

2 garlic cloves, crushed

1cm piece ginger, finely chopped

1 tsp tomato purée

1 tsp ground cumin

1 tsp garam masala

200g basmati rice

850ml vegetable stock

140g red lentils, washed and drained

200g bag spinach leaves, chopped

Handful mint leaves, chopped

8 peppers

Method

- Heat the oil in a large saucepan with a lid. Add the onion, garlic and ginger, then gently cook for 5 mins until softened. Stir in the tomato purée and spices, and cook for 1 min more. Add the rice, stir to coat, then pour in the stock. Bring to the boil, tip in the lentils, and cover with the lid and leave to cook over a low heat for 15 mins, until the lentils and rice are cooked. Stir through the spinach and mint (see tip below, if freezing).
- Use a sharp knife to slice the top off each pepper. Cut out the middle stalk and scoop out any seeds. Carefully trim the bottoms slightly so they stand upright, but the filling won't fall out. Fill each pepper with the rice mix and place the lid on top. Bake or wrap tightly in cling film or freezer bags and freeze.
- To cook, defrost peppers completely if frozen. Heat oven to 350 F. Place the peppers on a lightly greased baking tray and cook for 25-30 mins or until the peppers have softened. Serve with a green salad tossed with cucumber, herbs and a dollop of yogurt.

Jacket potatoes with home-baked beans

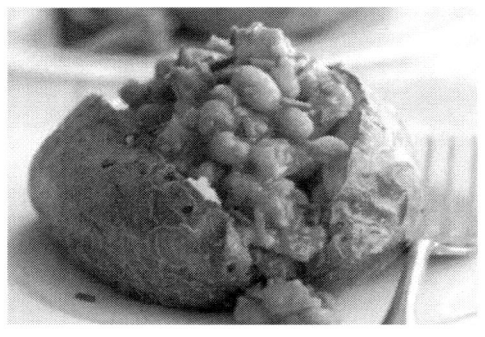

Makes 4 servings

237 calories per serving

Ingredients

    4 baking potatoes

    1 tbsp. sunflower oil

    1 carrot, diced

    1 celery stalk, diced

    400g can haricot beans, drained

    2 tomatoes, chopped

    1 tsp paprika - choose sweet or hot depending on taste

    1 tsp Worcestershire sauce

    2 tbsp. chopped chives, to serve

Method

- Heat oven to 3560 F. Scrub the potatoes and dry well, then prick in several places with a fork. Bake directly on the oven shelf for 1-1½ hours, until they feel soft when squeezed.
- After 30 mins, heat the oil in a pan and gently cook the carrot and celery for 10 mins until softened. Add the beans, tomatoes and paprika and cook gently for a further 5 mins until the tomatoes are softened and pulpy. Stir in 100ml water and the Worcestershire sauce, cook for a further 5 mins then cover and keep warm.
- Split open the potatoes and spoon in the beans. Scatter with chives and serve.

Acquacotta

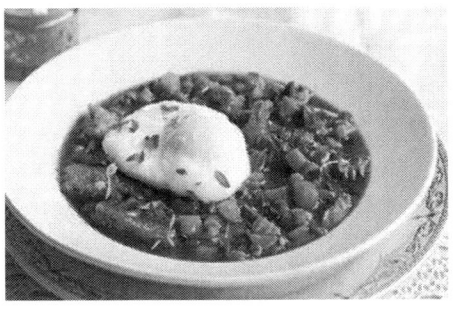

Makes 6 servings

239 calories per serving

Ingredients
    3 tbsp. olive oil

    3 celery sticks, chopped

    2 small carrots, chopped

    1 red onion, finely chopped

    2 garlic cloves, finely chopped

    2 tsp thyme leaves, plus extra to serve

    50g dried porcini mushrooms

    225g plum tomatoes, deseeded and chopped

    850ml chicken stock

    2 tbsp. chopped parsley

3 slices good crusty bread, toasted and torn into chunks

6 eggs

Method

- Heat the olive oil in a large saucepan and gently fry the celery, carrots, onion, garlic and thyme for 10-15 mins until softened. Meanwhile, cover the porcini with hot water and soak for 15 mins until softened and swollen. Drain the mushrooms, reserving the soaking liquid, and roughly chop. Add to the softened vegetables along with the soaking liquid and cook for another 5 mins.
- Stir in the tomatoes and cook for 10 mins until they begin to break down, then pour in the stock and bring to a gentle simmer.
- Poach the 6 eggs in a separate large saucepan of simmering water for 3-4 mins until set, then remove with a slotted spoon. Add the parsley and a little seasoning to the soup, and mix in the torn-up toasted bread. Divide the soup between 6 bowls and place an egg on top of each. Serve scattered with extra thyme.

Griddled vegetable & feta tart

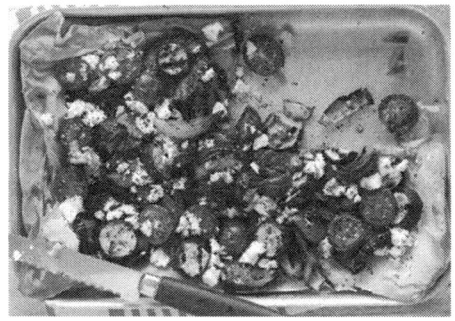

Makes 4 Servings

191 calories per serving

Ingredients
2 tbsp. olive oil

1 aubergine, sliced

2 courgette, sliced

2 red onion, cut into chunky wedges

3 large sheets filo pastry

10-12 cherry tomatoes, halved

Drizzle of balsamic vinegar

85g feta cheese, crumbled

1 tsp dried oregano

Large bag mixed salad leaves and low-fat dressing,

to serve

Method

- Heat oven to 400 F. Pop 33 x 23cm baking tray in the oven to heat up. Brush a griddle pan with about 1 tsp of the oil and griddle the aubergines until nicely charred, then remove. Repeat with the courgettes and onions, using a little more oil if you need to.
- Remove the tray from the oven and brush with a little oil. Brush a large sheet of filo with oil, top with another sheet, add a little more oil and repeat with the final sheet. Transfer the pastry to the hot tray, pushing it into the edges a little.
- Arrange the griddled veg on top, then season. Add the tomatoes, cut-side up, then drizzle on the vinegar and any remaining oil. Crumble on the feta and sprinkle with oregano. Cook for about 20 mins until crispy and golden. Serve with the dressed mixed salad leaves.

With two days of fasting, it will take you weeks to try all these recipes. But if you are looking for more options, search the internet for 5:2 recipes for fasting days. There are so many options out there that you will never get bored!

Chapter 6: What Foods Should I Keep in the House?

Want to know exactly what to keep on hand for the 5:2 diet fast days? This chapter will give you a good idea of things to have on hand in your pantry so that you will be prepared for your fasting days. The easiest way to stay full and not feel hungry on fasting days are to eat a lot of lean proteins, vegetables that are full of fiber, and to have plenty to drink, including water, tea, coffee, and seltzers, which have no calories. Here is a list of things to have on hand to make sure that you are prepared for your fast days.

Vegetables: Leafy, dark green vegetables are the best. They are very low in calories, have a lot of fiber, and are very filling. You can eat a lot of them without using a lot of your calories. Here are some vegetables that you can eat with their calorie count per serving so that you are aware of how much you can have:
Baby spinach: 12 calories per 1 cup serving of raw leaves

Arugula: 6 calories per cup of raw leaves

Swiss Chard: 7 calories per one cup of raw leaves

Watercress: 7 calories per 1 cup of raw leaves

Mustard Greens: 21 calories per 1 cup of raw leaves

Romaine Lettuce: 8 calories per one cup raw leaves

Iceberg lettuce: 8 calories per 1 cup raw leaves

As you can see, green, leafy vegetables contain a

great deal of punch for your calorie count. And, because they are full of fiber, they will keep you feeling full for a long time! Plus, they have a great many vitamins and minerals that will keep you healthy and happy, even on your fasting days.

Lean Proteins: Lean proteins are great because protein takes a longer time to digest, as compared to simple sugars and carbohydrates, so you will feel full longer. Some healthy proteins that you can eat on your fasting days include:

Lean pork tenderloin: 136 calories per 4 ounce serving

95% Lean Ground Beef: 148 calories per 3 ounce serving

Boneless, skinless chicken breast: 31 calories per 1 ounce

Roasted turkey breast without skin: 153 calories per 4 ounce serving

Tuna fillet: 157 calories per 3 ounce serving

Canned tuna: 194 calories in 1 6.5 ounce can

Tilapia fillet: 112 calories per 3 ounce serving

Salmon fillet: 177 calories per 3 ounce serving

1 Egg, large boiled: 78 calories

When preparing these meats, it is better to bake, roast, or grill them, rather than fry them, as frying will add calories to the count. Baking, roasting, or grilling without any oil will not.

Soups: There are many options for low-calorie servings of soup. You can either make them or buy them in a can. There are a few soup recipes in the last chapter that you can try, or look for low-calorie soup options at the grocery store. These can be very warming in the winter and are very satisfying.

Salads: Using salads with lean protein on top (such as boneless, skinless chicken breast) can make a delicious meal. Use vinegar and herbs as a dressing so as to not add any calories to your salad.

Snacks: Although snacking on the fast days may be frowned upon, having an idea or two will help you get through the day. Especially if you are doing several small meals throughout the day, you may find these useful to have on hand. They are also good snacks to use if you don't feel well during your first few fasting days. All these snacks have 50 or less calories per serving. The options here are many, so you will surely find something on this list that can satisfy you.

Dill pickles: 8 calories per pickle

2 egg whites: 48 calories

10 grapes: 35 calories

1 small pack raisins (think the box you ate in your lunch as a kid): 42 calories

8 ounces of Miso soup: 36 calories

½ grapefruit: 39 calories

10 green olives: 42 calories

1 cup air-popped popcorn without butter: 31 calories

10 cherries: 42 calories

7 celery stalks: 45 calories

1 light Babybel cheese: 40 calories

16 cherry tomatoes: 49 calories

10 spears of asparagus: 50 calories

1 small tangerine: 37 calories

50 blueberries: 39 calories

8 dry-roasted peanuts: 43 calories

1 small peach: 38 calories

1 Brazil nut: 32 calories

1 square of dark chocolate (1x1 inch) 27 calories

50 Blueberries: 39 calories

½ cup blackberries: 31 calories

½ cup raspberries: 32 calories

40 sugar snap peas: 44 calories

7 almonds: 49 calories

2 ounces cottage 1% low fat cottage cheese: 41 calories

This list gives you a great many options for a snack on the 5:2 diet without killing your meal plans. If you get the munchies, any of these are a good option. Just make sure to count the calories when you do so. You want to make sure to stay under your 500 calorie limit.

Drinks: As we have already discussed, staying hydrated is a necessary part of everyday life, but it can be even more helpful for you when you are on a fast day, as many people experience they signals of thirst as hunger instead. If you feel hungry during the day, first try drinking

something and see if this helps you feel fuller. Drinking regularly is necessary to be successful on fast days. Here are some drinks that you can keep in your pantry. None of them have any calories, so you can have as much as you want:
Water. If you struggle with drinking water, you can add a little flavor by adding a lemon wedge. 1/8 of a lemon, juiced in water, only adds 2 calories. If you dislike the blandness of water, this can make it more palatable for you.

Seltzer

Teas, any kind, including black tea, green tea, and herbal teas

Coffee, decaf or caffeinated. Remember, calories can add up if you put stuff in your coffee.

If you choose to add milk to your coffee or tea, remember that adding milk can add a few calories that need to be counted. 1 tablespoon of 1% milk adds 9 calories. 1 tablespoon of whole milk adds 17 calories. 1 tablespoon of skim milk adds 5 calories.

Now that you know what to keep on hand, it is important to note a couple things that will probably be off the list on your fast days. As mentioned previously, you can eat whatever you want on your fasting days as long as you keep your calorie count under the limit, but, to make that easier, you may want to avoid processed carbs, which are things like white bread, white rice, and pasta. Also, it will be easier to keep higher fat foods and sugars of the list on fast days, as the calories will add up very quickly. It may also be good to cut out many of the higher calorie fruits. Berries, however, are great for you, and there are several fruits listed on the snack list above that are good for you on fasting days. These can be especially helpful if you are craving some sugar or have a sweet tooth.

As you can see, there are a lot of options to stay satiated on your fasting days. Now that you know what to keep in your pantry, you are ready to make your grocery list and to get going! With all these options, staying happy and avoiding hunger should be easier than ever. You are now ready to start on the 5:2 diet.

Conclusion:

By now you should have a pretty good idea of how the 5:2 diet works and how to get started on this simple plan. The beauty of this diet is that you can eat normally for five days out of the week and only have to restrict calories for two. This makes it a lot easier to stick to, as you are not feeling constantly deprived. And because you can choose which days you are fasting, you can rearrange this diet to suit your changing schedule and lifestyle. You can plan to fast on days when it will not interfere with your family, friends, and your life. You can even go out to eat on this diet, so it will not adversely affect your life! So many people have found this diet much easier to stick to and have lost incredible amounts of weight because of it.

In this book, you have learned about what the 5:2 diet is, how to manage fast days, and have had all your questions about this diet answered. You have learned that the 5:2 diet is safe and can help improve such medical issues as insulin resistance, heart issues, high cholesterol, and even neurological disorders such as Alzheimer's and Parkinson's! With all these advantages, it is an amazing diet that people can stick to for a lifetime!

Since choosing foods for the fast days is the most difficult part of the 5:2 diet, this book gives you seven breakfast, seven lunch, and seven dinner recipes for use in starting to plan your food on the 5:2 diet. Also, several different food choices have been listed so that you know what to keep in your fridge so that you do not feel hungry on this diet.

Now that you have all the information you need to get started, what are you waiting for? By following the 5:2 diet plan, you can lose up to 85 pounds, feel and look great, and take care of your health! Good luck!

You may also like these books

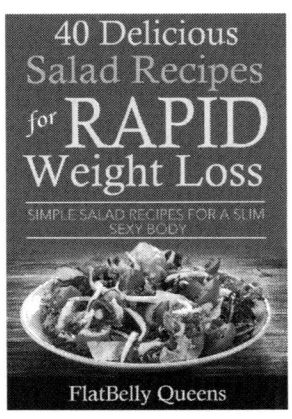

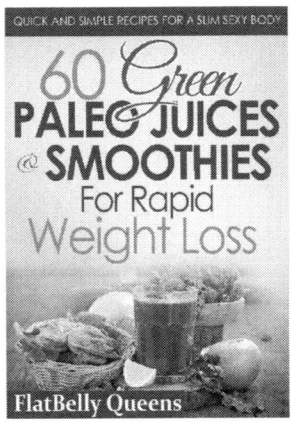

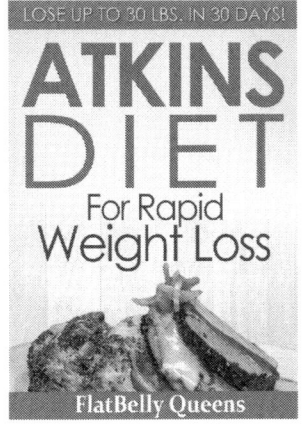

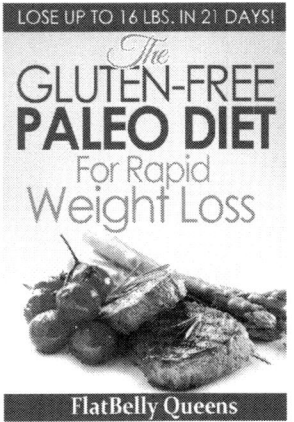

Printed in Great Britain
by Amazon